THE PERFECT MASSAGE

WELLNESS AT YOUR FINGERTIPS

Ingming Aberia

JULY 11, 2022
www.HealthBeautyAndFitness.today
New Jersey, USA

THE PERFECT MASSAGE

ISBN-13: 978-1500499075
ISBN-10: 1500499072
ASIN: ASIN: B00MGSSEMA

DEDICATION

To those whose lives were claimed by a novel virus on short or no notice at all—you are loved.

CONTENTS

DISCLAIMER

This information is provided "as is." The author, publishers and marketers of this information disclaim any loss or liability, either directly or indirectly as a consequence of applying the information presented herein, or in regard to the use and application of said information. No guarantee is given, either expressed or implied, regarding the merchantability, accuracy, or acceptability of the information.

Further, this information is not presented by a medical practitioner and is for educational and informational purposes only. The content is not intended to be a substitute for professional medical advice, diagnosis, or treatment. Always seek the advice of your physician or other qualified health provider with any questions you may have regarding a medical condition. Never disregard professional medical advice or delay in seeking it because of something you have read.

For any natural and/or dietary supplements we may recommend, please know further that statements related to them have not been evaluated by FDA and that the recommended product/s are/is not intended to "diagnose, treat, cure or prevent any disease."

1

INTRODUCTION: HOW TO GIVE THE PERFECT MASSAGE

Arguably, massage is among the best things to get after having a really stressful day. There is nothing that can believe the body of pains and aches like a good massage can.

It has been proven that touch therapy is among the best methods for stress relief since it not only invigorates the body, but the soul and mind as well. A massage helps to clear the passage towards the body and mind functioning harmoniously by unifying these two elements.

A massage in physical terms will induce good blood circulation and relaxation. Also, the motion created by the massage induces toxins to be excreted from the body.

Individuals visit massage therapists every once in a while to enjoy the experience of having a good massage. Another awesome thing is learning how to give a good massage to others. Just think how nice it would be to be able to give your loved one a massage and effectively reliever her of any pain she might be experiencing in her joints and muscles.

There are numerous ways to give a massage. From a strict sense, there are over 30 kinds of massages that are formerly recognized all around the world. So, which one should you choose to learn? Which one do you want to use?

This article provides some basic tips for how you can execute massages properly over various prominent body parts. We will be discussing how to best massage the head, face, chest, neck, arm, hand, leg, foot and back.

Back Massage

The back is one of the major body parts that normally needs to be massaged. Usually, the back hurts due to the person's body structure and posture. An individual who works in a chair all day certainly will feel stress on her or his back after working hard all day. Someone with a large stomach is also likely to experience back pain due to all the extra weight that must be supported.

When you are getting ready to give a back massage, keep in mind that there are three areas that will most benefit from having a back massage. They are the hip bones, shoulder blades and spine. Smooth circular presses can be employed along the person's shoulder blades. This will help to relax the muscles that are in that area. You can use smooth straight slides for relaxing muscles in a person's spine area. Slow circular presses can be used to massage the hip bones.

Leg and Foot Massage

Every day, the average individual walks thousands of steps. People who work in hard shoes or high heels will have foot pain when they are finished working. They could use a good foot massage. Having a great foot massage performed will provide the foot with better blood circulation. Stroking with an upward motion starting at the ankle up the leg relieves tension coming from the individual's blood vessels. Another good way to relieve foot stress is to rotate the ankle. The soles of the feet should also be gently massaged by providing the painful areas with circular presses.

Arm and Hand Massage

When smooth stroke patterns are applied along the hands and arms, this induces better blood circulation. The arms should also be rotated using a circular motion for loosening the joints. To avoid further pain, always massage the hands gently.

Chest and Neck Massage

Bad posture can result in chest and neck pain. Smooth downward strokes can be made, starting below the ear up to the shoulder. This can help with relieving neck tension. Employ circular motion double-handed finger presses in the back of the neck area.

Head and Face Massage

The face can also be massaged. In fact, a head and face massage can be very relaxing. The temples are one of the better head and face areas to massage. Provide some pressure as you press the temples using a circular motion. For added comfort, massage the forehead and cheekbones as well.

So those are some basic tips for giving an entire body massage. In the end, massage execution and technical know-how are quite important. However, what really counts is the willingness and love to provide your loved one with relief from her or his body pains.

2

DO-IT-YOURSELF MASSAGE: HOW IT CAN IMPROVE YOUR WELL-BEING

The Practice of Self Massage

In ancient times, self-massage was one of the most popular methods of healing various ailments. Together with infusions or mixtures made from herbs with healing powers, self-massage was recommended by doctors to their patients as an effective way to alleviate pains.

This practice is also used today. There were also several studies that showed beyond any doubt the benefits of self-massage for the overall health, as well as for specific medical conditions.

It is well-known that the human touch has a very big importance in the development of children. Even adults who don't get their daily fix of human touch are more prone to developing depression than those who benefit from the touch of other persons.

Self-massage has a broad range of benefits. It improves metabolism, speeds up the digestion process and helps eliminating waste more effectively. It also improves the blood circulation and relaxes the muscles. All these physical effects have their correspondent in psychical ones. The individual will feel more relaxed and even smarter, given the fact that massaging various centers in the body helps improving focus and clears the mind.

The biggest advantage of self-massage is that it can be practiced virtually anywhere: in the bus, at work, while shopping or while waiting in line for various errands. It can also be performed while watching your favorite TV show. You can do it with or without your clothes on, as long as you find yourself a comfortable position.

This portion of the report covers a basic massage technique for hands, shoulders, and feet. You can use it for alleviating various pains in your body, so read carefully and give it a try.

Hands Massage

As you probably know already, we use our hands a lot each day. From cooking to eating, from driving to operating a computer, everything requires us to use the hands. They could benefit from a relaxing massage, so here's what you can do:

Start by stroking one of your hands with the other one, using gentle, circular moves. If you want, you can use some hand cream for a better feeling. The next step is to squeeze your hand, then move towards each finger and press it gently from the base to the tip. Pull and stretch your fingers one by one, then repeat the procedure with the other hand.

With your thumb, massage the palm of your hand, following a circular pattern. Work it from the base of the fingers to the wrist, making sure to insist on the joints and tendons.

Feet Massage

Feet are very important. Ancient Chinese believed that the entire human body with all its organs is represented on the foot. By massaging those zones, your organs will also benefit, thus helping you improve your well-being.

For an effective self-massage of the feet, you need to rest one of the feet on the opposite leg, then use both your hands to massage your sole with gentle moves up and down, insisting on those areas where you fell tension or pain.

Toes need a special attention. Take them one by one and rub them slowly with your fingers. When you are done, apply some nourishing cream or lotion on your feet and relax for a while to allow the skin to absorb the nutrients and the moisture.

Shoulders Massage

If you spend a lot of time at your desk every day, you probably know already how painful and tensed your neck and shoulders can become at the end of such a demanding day. You can alleviate neck pains and relieve the tension in your back and in your shoulders by applying a special self-massage during your lunch break or whenever you have a spare moment in your work.

Start the massage by sitting in the right position at your desk. Mold your palms to the natural curves of your shoulders, then apply gentle strokes as you glide from the back of your neck towards the shoulders, arms and elbows. Repeat the strokes for about 3-4 minutes.

Grab and pinch the upper part of your shoulders and start to apply gentle squeezing while you more up and down. You can also massage your face, as well as your scalp.

It's true that a massage therapy applied by a professional can be extremely effective, but it is also true that in the absence of the therapist we can do little things like self-massaging our hands, feet, and shoulders in order to improve our well-being and to put ourselves into a more cheerful and relaxed mood. Self-massage is very powerful and besides it is absolutely free and easy to do pretty much everywhere. Take advantage of it and enjoy your days more.

It's in your power to feel better, all you need to do for this is to make good use of your hands.

3

PREGNANCY AND MASSAGE

The Basics of Pregnancy and Massage

Pregnancy is among the most fulfilling and rewarding states that a woman can be in. However, it is often also one of the more painful experiences she can endure, given all the dramatic changes that an expectant mother goes through during her pregnancy.

An expectant mother, during her pregnancy, may experience:

- Her intestines, stomach and diaphragm being pushed up by her uterus
- Her digestive system becoming displaced
- Weight gain that stresses the joints and bones
- Skin discoloration, rashes, and breakouts
- Increased urination
- Oxygen consumption by the lungs is increased by more than 10%
- Blood flow inside the kidney increases 35%
- Blood volume is increased by the heart by as much as 50%

The therapeutic practice of massage during pregnancy can help to relieve many of the above common pains and help to reduce the chances of them occurring and sometimes even prevent them from developing at all. Massage therapy can also improve general body tone and circulation, enhance joint and muscle functions and relieve mental fatigue.

Pregnancy and Massage Therapy

These days massage therapy that is provided to pregnant women, which is referred to more commonly as prenatal massage, has been a practice that recently has been developing quite rapidly in the United States. The field has been attracting many professionals like childbirth educators, midwives, obstetricians, and delivery nurses.

This field's popularity is due to more women focusing on wellness while pregnant. Since most women these days postpone having children until they have stable careers and relationships, they search for alternative methods that can help with alleviating pain that is experienced during a traditional pregnancy.

Prenatal Massage Benefits

Massage therapy can reduce the uncomfortable and stressful experiences that occur during pregnancy. Specifically, it can help with:

- Relieving soreness and stiffness following childbirth Realigning the pelvis after giving birth
- Speeding up the healing process after cesarean birth or during postpartum recovery
- Increasing milk production
- Having an easier childbirth
- Relieving sinus congestion
- Lessening sciatic pain
- Reducing feet and hands swelling
- Assisting proper posture
- Relieving back and neck pain caused by imbalance and muscle weakness
- Decreasing insomnia
- Eliminating waste products via the lymphatic and circulatory systems
- Reducing stress to the heart
- Increasing circulation
- Having better sleep and relaxing
- Increasing muscle flexibility
- Stabilizing hormone levels
- Increasing oxygen and nutrients to the fetus cells and mother
- Relieving sciatica, stick necks, edema, sore feet, backaches, and headaches
- Alleviating tension, tightness, stiffness, and muscle cramping.

In addition to all the physical benefits that massage therapy offers during a pregnancy, receiving soothing human touch can feel very good to expectant mothers. Also, according to a Miami School of Medicine study, massage therapy can reduce stress hormones inside the body.

This study showed that human touch is very important for a mother's physical and emotional wellbeing, given that she must adapt to her new body. An expectant mother's body is changed, stressed, and challenged in many ways, no matter what her personal conditions are. Prenatal massage provides a pregnant woman with special attention. This nurtures the baby as well that is developing inside her.

A pregnant woman can be given a massage by her husband, a relative or friend. However, to receive the full benefits that prenatal massage can provide, it is highly recommended that the pregnant woman sees an experienced massage therapist who has been certified in pregnancy, labor, and postpartum massage.

Is Prenatal Massage Therapy Right for You?

Pregnancy and massage, for most mothers, is an ideal match. However, before giving a massage, the professional massage therapist discusses potential personal problems or complications of the pregnancy with the expectant mother.

Massage therapists generally do not provide prenatal massages to women with conditions like contagious illnesses, malignant conditions, vomiting, diarrhea, pre-eclampsia, morning sickness, abdominal pain, high blood pressure, unusual pain, blood discharge, heavy water, diabetes, or fever.

Also, any of a pregnant woman's body parts with raised or distended varicose veins, local infection sites, inflammation, sores, bruises, or skin rashes shouldn't be massaged.

There are several different ways that pregnancy massage can be performed.

The pregnant woman might lie on either her belly or side. There are pillows that have been designed especially for pregnant women. They make is possible for them to lie on their stomachs flat, no matter how far along in their pregnancies they are.

A prenatal massage can last from 20 minutes to 60 minutes. It depends on the amount of discomfort that a pregnant woman is experiencing. During a pregnant woman's second trimester, it is strongly recommended that she see her massage therapist once a week at least to receive treatment.

It is a very challenging, miraculous, and wonderful experience to introduce a new life to the world. Parental massage can help to make your pregnancy be a much more enjoyable and comfortable experience.

4

THE ART OF CHILD AND INFANT MESSAGE

For centuries people have massaged children and babies. In terms of healing arts from the world's traditional cultures, it's considered among the most effective. Although child and infant massage doesn't yet have worldwide acceptance, it's an instinctive act that a parent provides to her or his child.

Over the past decade, child massage has grown tremendously in terms of popularity in the United States as well as other areas of the world. Today, many grandparents, friends, guardians, mothers, and fathers are looking for instructors who can guide and educate them in the art of child and infant massage.

Massage can help all babies, however for infants it is especially beneficial.

According to some infant message research, massaging infants helps with increasing premature infant weight gain by as much as 45%. Also, touching an infant and holding a baby on your chest has been proven to shorten a baby's hospital stay.

Benefits of Child and Infant Massage

Child and infant massage are critical for developing and improving psychological, physical, and emotional characteristics of your infant or child.

Relaxation. You might think that the life of an infant just revolves around sleeping, eating and the changing of diapers. However, they are caught in an existence that involves constant changes. What this means is that they have gone from being inside the comfortable and warm womb of the mother, into a world where everything is new to them.

Even children and infants are prone to getting stress. Our fast-paced world makes adults tend to forget about relaxation. Children and infants notice this, and as a result they don't learn how to relax either.

The muscles are eased by massages. This leads to relaxation. Massaging your child regularly will help him or her learn relaxation fundamentals, and eventually he or she will relax all on their own.

Parent's Awareness. Given that the adult is going to be involved on a regular basis helping the baby to relax, she or he will learn to understand what the needs of the child are. Also, it's an excellent way of developing a bond at an early age with the infant.

Relief. Your infant or child experiencing pain is normal. The more common discomforts that baby experience are teething pain, gas and spasm. There are certain massage techniques that help with easing emotional stress, toning the digestive system, relieving pain associated with teething, dispersing gas, easing muscle spasms, and relieving pain. When you message an infant, you may also buy soothing oils. The aroma can help with calming your child down.

Stimulation. The muscles of a child can get tense and might need to be massaged to relax them. However, the muscles might be loose as well. Massage can stimulate them.

Child massage helps with stimulating the muscles as well as stimulating other body systems as well. For example, massage helps with digestion. This in turn can help with easing constipation symptoms.

Usually, infants have cold feet or hands. When this occurs, it is due to poor circulation. This can be countered by massaging the feet or hands until they become warm. Massage helps with stimulating blood flow in an infant.

Parent-Child Bonding. A parent and child bonding is a continual process that starts an early age until the infant becomes older. Child or infant massage encourages strong and unique interaction between child and parent.

If you get into the habit of massaging your child daily, she or he will come to expect the message on schedule. You can either massage your child after they wake up, before they go to sleep, or after a bath.

Be sure the room that you are going to be massaging your child in is comfortable and warm for both of you. Keep in mind that premature infants are not able to regulate their own body temperatures. Therefore, it is very important that the room is set to a comfortable temperature.

There have been several studies that have shown how infants prefer massages done with oil. Most massage therapists recommend vegetable or plant oil or aromatherapy that offer a gentle scent. Be sure to not use other mineral- based oil since they are not absorbed easily.

The first couple of weeks in a baby's life might appear to be all about mother-infant interaction and breastfeeding. Many fathers end up feeling left out.

Therefore, infant massage could be a nice way for him to bond with his new baby in addition to alleviating certain body pains that the infant might have.

Infant massage might only ease pain on a temporary basis. However, it's the most loving and natural act a parent can provide a child when he or she is young.

5

DEEP TISSUE MASSAGE BENEFITS

Today, life has become more of a complicated hassle. People have become too busy working so hard that often they have no time at all to take good care of themselves. The saddest part is that one can never fully realize they are living such a lifestyle until it's too late. The issue is that the problem is not easily recognized until the body is stressed to the point where the individual is plagued with diseases or other health and medical conditions.

For instance, when the body's muscles are stressed, oxygen flow is hampered. At the same time, essential nutrients needed by the body are wasted instead of being absorbed. This then leads to inflammation and accumulation of toxins in muscles making it more painful to move around.

The interesting thing to note is that this does not happen only to the elderly. People of all ages too are vulnerable to the effects associated with body stress. It doesn't really matter how strong you think your body is, but if you mistreat it, there surely will be some negative effects.

Our bodies need some pampering occasionally. The body, if overworked, cannot be as productive as you would want it to be. The good thing is that there are options that you could take up to combat tension and stress.

And one such way is the deep tissue massage.

The deep tissue massage is a technique which concentrates on and targets the inner muscle tissue layers of the body. The main objective of this massaging technique is to lower tension in the body by slowly stroking and putting pressure on certain contracted parts of the body.

Deep tissue massage is yet another technique that targets and concentrates on the inner layers of the muscle tissue. Its main objective is to loosen body tension through the application of pressure using slow finger strokes on contracted areas of the body.

The deep tissue massage technique is because of years of study and caters well to the relaxation needs of a tense body. As such, instead of getting a plain body massage, this massage option promises to be more beneficial.

As this massage technique is more centered and specific, you may experience some soreness during and after the procedure. However, this feeling may disappear within a day or two; that is if it was done in the right way-pressure is applied across the grain of the muscle.

There are several benefits to having a deep tissue massage done. One gets to loosen muscle tissues, there is improved oxygen and blood circulation and toxins in the muscles are released. However, it is essential that you drink plenty of water before and after having the procedure since it will help in flushing out the toxins.

Toxin build-up in the body obviously has negative effects on the body. Most of the times, symptoms may not be so obvious, but you may start feeling bad when the problem becomes a major one. It is therefore important that you closely monitor your lifestyle and how it affects your overall well-being and health.

Furthermore, deep tissue massage targets those deeply seated hints of tension in your body. As such, many consider it as both a therapeutic and corrective procedure that addresses issues that are not easily addressed by a simple massage.

The movements and techniques of deep tissue massaging are quite like those of a Swedish massage. However, with this option, there is more pressure being put on the muscles. Such intense pressures on specific areas help in releasing muscle adhesions known as chronic muscle knots. While the procedure may be a bit uncomfortable and unsettling, it is worth it. The good thing is that you could always request the masseuse to lessen the pressure if you feel it's too much.

While you are promised of great results, achieving them will not happen immediately or after a single session. Yes, you may feel much better, but if your intention is to correct a problem, then more sessions will be necessary. Just as it is with any treatment, commitment and patience must be virtues you embrace. Also, you will need to have faith that the treatment will do something towards rectifying your condition.

At the same time, it is very important that you consider who is handling the procedure on you. Do they have the capacity and knowledge to do it right? Research on different institutions that are known to offer the best of these services. Or else, you will be putting yourself at risk of getting injured or harmed.

The deep tissue massage option is indeed a viable option for one seeking to overcome the negative stress effects. Nonetheless, for the procedure to bear the kind of results you seek, it needs to be coupled with a lifestyle change. If you are continuously going back to your old habits, then deep tissue massage will not work for you no matter how often you are going for treatment.

6

ABOUT AROMATHERAPY AND MASSAGE

What Is Aromatherapy and Massage and Why Is It Called 'The Perfect Combination to Harmonized Therapy'?

What is aromatherapy? It is a therapeutic form of healing making use of several aromas derived from pure leaves, herbs, flowers, and other plant extracts. These extracts are usually in the form of oils which are therapeutic when inhaled and/or applied on one's skin.

Different oils have different applications. For instance, essential oils are never meant to be applied in pure form as they are known to cause a burning, redness, or irritating sensation. Oils like grape seed, almond, and jojoba oil, also known as carrier oils, are usually meant to be mixed.

It is important to note that the use of a specific oil type successively for 12 weeks and over may not be as effective as the skin will develop resistance towards it.

When it comes to the putting away of aromatherapy oils, storage in a cool and dry place is essential for these oils to preserve their efficiency. It is also advisable to store them in dark bottles that will not allow light to penetrate through as it deteriorates them, lowering their effectiveness over time. Properly stored oils will last for years.

Aromatherapy and massaging complement each other very well. The massage procedure is well known for its effectiveness in the loosening of muscle contractions, improvement of oxygen and blood circulation and release of toxins. As such, the use of aromatherapy oils when getting massage will no doubt be beneficial to the patient.

Massage and aromatherapy easily affect one's autonomic nervous system. It considerably calms the flight and fight response, reducing stress hormone levels in our bodies. Studies have proven that people with significantly lower stress levels are less prone to diseases and recover faster and easily from ailments or other health issues.

This harmonized therapy is widely embraced and used by many healthcare facilities all over the world. It has proven to be a procedure that has considerably improved many patients' quality of life. As such, it is now being offered to cancer patients as a supportive therapy form.

To support this, London's Marie Curie Cancer Care conducted research on 103 cancer patients. The patients either received an aromatherapy massage or a plain massage. The results showed that the patients who got aromatherapy massages done on them showed significantly lowered levels of anxiety when compared to those who got a plain massage done. Other things noted were the improvements in these patients' physical comfort, quality of life and disposition.

In conclusion, the research proved that aromatherapy oils improve the psychological and physical well-being of patients while at the same time improving their physical comfort from the massage they received. At the same time, the results were combined with touch therapy benefits boosted by the effectiveness of aromatherapy.

Not only has aromatherapy combined with massage proven to be beneficial to cancer patients but it also helps people with disabilities- in this case learning disabilities. Touch and smell senses play a big role in this area.

The human's olfactory system is directly connected to the body's limbic system- the part of the brain that deals with emotions. At the same time, smell and touch senses are seemingly less complicated when compared to sight and hearing. As such, creating a form of communication that maximizes on smell and touch is easier for individuals with learning disabilities.

Learning disability individuals are usually characterized by monotonous actions and stereotypical behaviors that have no purpose- characteristics synonymous with their sense impairment. Through massage and aromatherapy, these characteristics significantly lower.

The combined procedure causes the person to start becoming aware of their body and helps in building a tolerance to touch. It helps as it makes the person less inclined to self-stimulation. As such, the patient can focus on something else other than him/herself. The initial manifestations are the patient's capacity to start interacting with his/her therapist.

Furthermore, athletes can benefit from the aromatherapy massage too. For some time now, this procedure has been of training for many athletes. It not only enhances performance but also improves an athlete's recovery rate. For serious athletes, aromatherapy massages are a norm and have them done before and even after every activity or game.

Certainly, massage and aromatherapy can do wonders especially if done carefully and in the right way.

Since combining both aromatherapy and massage has proven to be extremely effective in relieving some health conditions, health professionals are required to go through several years of training. Aromatherapy oil uses are powerful, endless and should not be underrated.

7

ACUPRESSURE PRESSURE POINT THERAPY-WHAT IS IT AND HOW DOES IT WORK?

In general, pressure point therapy, involves pressing certain points on the body. They are scattered across the body. Usually, they are found on the knuckles, limbs, palms, and fingers. The pressure point that needs to be focused on depends mainly on the type of illness the individual is feeling. Acupressure, most of the time, is performed to promote good health and relieve pain and stress.

Acupressure is like acupuncture, the traditional Chinese way of healing. It also originated around 5,000 years ago in China. However, instead of needles being used to treat a specific disease, in its place a specific amount of pressure gets applied.

Acupressure in the United States is largely used for relaxation and relief. However, in China, it gets used as a kind of first aid. Acupressure is applied on individuals who are suffering with hangovers, headaches, sore muscles, and colds.

It is easy to learn the acupressure technique. For your first few treatments, you may need to visit a specialist. As you get familiar with this process, then you can progress to doing acupressure to others and for yourself.

Acupressure touches on the ancient Chinese beliefs of energies, chakras, and chees. Acupressure is known for facilitating vital energy flow within the body. The ancient Chinese medicine believes that when the body's energy flow is hindered in some way, sickness will follow soon after.

Acupressure is charged with releasing the blocked energies of an individual.

The principle is followed also by acupuncture therapy, acupressure's counterpart. The acupressure technique involves stimulating the acupoints.

These are the specific energy points of the body. They are called energy channels as well.

The acupressure technique is the act that involves firmly pressing the points. While the practitioner does this, the body's energy starts flowing again towards those parts that are experiencing discomfort or illness. The results in a way of healing that is gradual but very effective.

Acupressure doesn't use any needles or tools. A hand massage is used by pressing specific body parts manually. This method, scientifically speaking, might help to release endorphins from the body. These are natural painkillers that exist inside the body.

How long an acupressure treatment will last can vary greatly, anywhere from minutes all the way up to an hour. It depends on how sick or well the patient is. It may be done either in a lying or sitting position. Some therapists need patients to dress in just a towel to perform full body therapy.

Every specific body point corresponds to a specific illness. For example, back pain is addressed through pressing that specific body point, which is located behind your knees. Pressing the body point that is on top of the foot, on the other hand, provides relief for migraines.

Usually, pressure is applied for approximately 3 to 10 seconds. However, in many cases, it might be longer than that. If necessary, it can repeatedly be done. The relief is usually instant. However, if the problem exists still, or if the severity level doesn't go down at least, then the acupressure isn't considered to be effective. For you it may not be effective for your specific ailment or on that day.

Acupressure therapy's overall impact is loosening up and absolute relaxation. There might be minimal muscle aching. However, it shouldn't be so strong that it is painful.

The initial therapists' visits are usually three to eight sessions. After that, it should be possible for you to figure out whether acupressure is effective for you. For stress management, it required to have a monthly or weekly series of treatments for best results.

Many people have given acupressure a try and have been pleased with the results. Even the pains that have been caused by nausea and surgical operations are also relieved. It also helps with other body conditions like morning sickness, motion sickness and sinusitis.

To experience the best of what acupressure therapy can provide, your first step will be locating a good therapist to go to. However, unfortunately now there aren't any acupressure licensing programs. Try getting recommendations from family members and friends instead who have experience with acupressure. That should be a great place for you to start finding a good therapist you can go to.

If you would like to ease the pain from out of your body without having to use any chemicals or medicines, acupressure therapy is something that is worth trying out. Experience the benefits it offers for yourself and see if the better options are doing things the natural way. Insert chapter seven text here.

8

REFLEXOLOGY—THE BENEFITS THAT COME WITH THE PRESSURE POINT THERAPY

For those who are interested in learning more about pressure point therapy, it's important to know that reflexology has been enjoying great popularity because of its benefits. In reflexology, physical pressure is applied to a variety of targeted areas on a person's feet and hands by a reflexologist. It is very relaxing and promotes an alternative way of natural healing.

The belief behind this form of natural healing is that certain areas on a person's palms and the soles of their feet correlate to other specific organs and areas throughout that person's body.

Reflexologists use their fingers to apply the pressure to each of these zones. When specific pressure is applied to these areas, it is said that it will help to create more positive health in the body that is being targeted.

Records show that reflexology was made use of in early India and China, although the initial origin of reflexology is not known. It is believed that we now have this natural healing art thanks to someone from one of these countries.

A doctor named William H. Fitzgerald, who specialized in Otolaryngology, was the person who introduced reflexology to the US in the early 1900s. Reflexology as we know it today was improved by him with his introduction of "zone therapy." Dr. Fitzgerald discerned that applying a certain amount of pressure to a person's palms and foot soles would affect the health of other corresponding areas of the body in a positive way.

Not long after, it was learned by a physical therapist by the name of Eunice Ingham that applying pressure to a person's foot provided even greater benefits than applying pressure to hands does. Ms. Ingham was able to map out each zone on the foot in detail to show the areas of the body that each zone corresponded to.

She was able to discern that what goes on in a person's toes mirror their neck and head health. In addition, she learned that a person's heart, lungs and chest are mirrored by the ball of their feet. The right side of a person's body is reflected by their left foot, and the left side of their body is reflected in their right foot.

Reflexology is considered to work much like Chinese medicine does. For example, a person's body is believed to be brimming with energy in the art of Chinese medicine. Further, if the body's energy flow is blocked in any way, it will cause disease to come about.

Research shows that there are approximately 7,000 nerve endings located within a human's foot. Imagine a person's nervous system as a computer, and a person's foot as the computer's keyboard. By pressing certain areas of the foot (or the buttons on a body's keyboard), it is believed that it will stop the energy blockage in the body and help the energy to flow properly again.

Reflexology is believed to work much the same way that acupuncture does. There is one main difference though, and this comes about due to treatment being given to more body parts in acupuncture. In reflexology, treatment involves only a person's hand and feet.

Endorphins and chemicals are believed to be released in the body when the right type of pressure is applied to hands and feet. This release is known to be the body's way of dealing with pain naturally. The chemicals and endorphins help decrease a person's stress levels. Today's current medical research also shows this to be the case.

A reflexologist typically begins a session with a client by asking them several questions. They will need to know of their health condition now and the lifestyle they lead. They will also ask the client about any previous illnesses they have had in the past or currently have.

The client will then be asked to remove their socks and shoes and sit back in a comfortable chair that reclines. Some reflexologists will ask their client to lay down on a cushioned table instead. Based on information shared by the client, the reflexologist may then discuss the areas of the foot they will be working on.

Next, they will first give the client's foot a rubdown. This is said to help warm the foot up for the work to come. Any sensitivity or knotted areas in the feet will show the reflexologist that energy is blocked in the areas of the body that reflect the affected areas of the feet.

Further work on the feet will show the reflexologist whether other areas of the body needed to be targeted. One of these sessions can sometimes last as long as 60 minutes or be as quick as only 30 minutes.

For best results, a client should have a reflexology session at least once per week. It is a good idea to pay close attention to the exact areas of the foot the reflexologist works on during a session. This knowledge will allow a client to work on those areas themselves while at home.

The art of reflexology is considered to an excellent alternative medicine for natural healing. But despite its popularity, it is not meant to be a substitution for any treatments that are needed by a medical professional. Reflexology is a supplement that helps to assist the process of healing. Anyone who has an interest in the benefits of natural healing should book a reflexology appointment to see how it will benefit them.

9

SHIATSU-PRESSURE POINT THERAPY THAT IS REVOLUTIONARY

The Japanese people have their very own pressure point therapy and line of massage. The Chinese people have their acupuncture, and the people of Japan have their shiatsu. The term shiatsu originates from the Japanese words-shi (meaning finger) and atsu (meaning pressure).

Shiatsu in Japan is a form of hands-on healing. In the west, especially in the United States, this is the closest thing there is to Chiropractic massages. It follows anatomy and physiology ideology. The thumbs, palms and fingers are the major body parts that are used when giving a shiatsu massage. Knees and elbows are not used.

Japanese Shiatsu practitioner are required to be licensed to perform this kind of therapy. They are referred to as Shiatsupractors. Shiatsu was introduced to North America by Tokujiro Namikoshi. He came from a shiatsupractors line and was trained properly in the craft.

When searching for a good shiatsu practitioner in the U.S., be sure to check to see if the person is certified by the American Bodywork Therapy Association (ABTA). In case you need additional verification, the association's office is in New Jersey.

Shiatu's essence is to heal and to diagnose. Irregularities of the body are detected with the fingers, thumbs, and palms. These can be tended to properly once they have been diagnosed.

The detection process, or implementing the analyzing skills of a practitioner, is the hardest part when it comes to learning Shiatsu. The training focuses on this.

People who would like to have natural healing done by having a shiatsu massage don't need to have been diagnosed previously of earlier illnesses or pains.

Shiatsu has the capability of healing and knowledge all at once. In addition, shiatsu is capable also of preventing diseases. Prevention, it has often been said, is better than the cure always.

One shiatsu session lasts for approximately one hour. How many sessions are necessary for optimal healing depends on how severe your illness is. For problems that are acute, having somewhere between 4 to 8 sessions is sufficient. Acute problems include stress and headaches. Chronic conditions such as back pain often require treatments over a longer period.

Just like any other kind of treatment procedure, the first step is always noting one's medical history. Practitioners want to be informed about their patient's diets and lifestyles. This helps them with each session they work on the patient.

The client is always fully clothed and lying down during a shiatsu session. The pressing and massaging is done by the practitioner with the client on the floor on a mat. The first touch goes to the abdominal area. This is thought to be where the tension in the body starts.

The idea is to allow energy to flow through the body. The main goal of pressing is facilitating the energy of the body to freely move. Healing is initiated when the energy is flowing nicely.

Shiatsu isn't a traditional form of massage. Many other kinds of techniques are involved, including stretching, rotating, and holding. Rubbing and kneading are used as well. Other kinds of shiatsu massage use the feet also.

Shiatsu massage provides an overall relaxing effect to the body. Patients, however, might feel a bit strange due to how the body reacts to it. Your stomach might start gurgling or tension could cause sudden shudders. These are normal, however, and you don't need to worry.

Following a shiatsu session, different people have various body reactions. Some individuals might feel sleepy. Others could feel invigorated. It is expected that you will feel exuberant following a session. This feeling could even last for one to two weeks following treatment.

Having shiatsu massages on a regular basis can help protect you against common illness and ensure good health. It is highly recommended for individuals having problems with coping with their stress daily. People who have muscular aches and tension will benefit the most because they can get outright relief.

Shiatsu in general is good for your body. However, if you have rashes or open wounds, avoid treatment. Don't go to a session if you've had an operation recently or have a tendency for getting blood clots. These situations could pose health risks for you.

People with abdominal illnesses or who are pregnant, in general shouldn't attend shiatsu sessions until their health has been restored. However, those who do attend sessions shouldn't eat for two hours at least prior to the treatment.

Shiatsu is a great option for individuals wanting to rid themselves of stress. Try shiatsu if you are wanting to do this the natural way and avoid taking pills. This might be the pressure point therapy you've been searching for all along.

10

KINESIOLOGY AND MASSAGE—WHAT YOU NEED TO KNOW

Kinesiology studies how people's bodies respond and move to messages that the brain sends. The terms come from the root word kinetics. The literal meaning is having a deep understanding of movement. In alternative medicine the most popular application for kinesiology is as a kind of massage therapy involving monitoring the muscles to figure out what might be imbalanced or wrong in an individual's body.

The Kinesiology technique scrutinizes stress reactions very carefully that might be unresolved in a person's body. The Kinesiology practitioner from this would help the body naturally heal with assistance from procedures like massage.

The Development of Kinesiology

Frequently Kinesiology is viewed as a branch of chiropractics. It combines with chi energy, the ancient Chinese principle that is demonstrated frequently in acupuncture. Muscle monitoring or biofeedback is used by Kinesiology to guide practitioners when massage therapy is being used.

How Kinesiology Works

A normal and healthy nervous system is designed creatively for adapting to environmental changes and self-regulation. However, there also can be times when the body is unable to adapt well. This results in stress in the muscles. Then Kinesioogists look to see if there are muscle stress patterns to try to figure out what the cause of the problems are and see if they can be fixed.

What Can Kinesiology Treat?

Kinesiology can treat a wide array of ailments through stimulating energies of the body as well as tapping into the body's hidden potential for healing itself. Many ailments stem from body imbalances. Therefore, Kinesiology can help to cure or treat many of different disorders, both mental and physical. Some of the numerous health problems that Kinesiology can treat include psychomotor difficulties, nutritional deficiencies, nervous disorders, stress, emotional problems, allergies, and muscular disorders.

How Kinesiology Is Practiced

Usually, a Kinesiology practitioner gets the patient's health history. Then the patient lies on a massage table while still fully clothed. The practitioner then performs several tests that involve the patient. The trials used will depend on what the patient's specific health problems are. Some tests that might be part of a Kinesiology session include:

Physical Test. The Kinesiology practitioner tests the integrity of the patient's neuromucular system. The patient is asked to manipulate an arm or leg in
specific ways. Then the patient holds the position, while the practitioner places mild pressure on the leg or arm.

Chemical Test. The practitioner tests the patient's reaction to specific foods or allergies by putting small quantities of the substance into the body. Then the Kinesiologist examines the reaction of the body of observing the relationship of the muscles to each other as well as the associated organs.
Mental Test. The practitioner gets the patient to think about specific feelings or objects while monitoring the muscles. During this session, certain stress reactions or imbalances are watched.

Kinesiology uses a wide array of different techniques, including nutritional counseling, trigger and reflex points, massages that emphasizes the body, hypertonic muscle release, acupressure and homeopathic remedies like emotional release, lymphatic massage, and aromatherapy.

Has Kinesiology Been Medically Proven?

There are many nervous system ailments that can potentially influence muscle strength. There isn't a lot of scientific research, however, that backs the Kinesiology philosophy up. It is seen to be a health practice that instead of using medical principles uses an energy model. Despite this, there have been significant numbers of patients who have undergone professional Kinesiology therapy and provided strong testimonials regarding the relief they have experienced following their Kinesiology sessions in addition to large improvements to their overall well-being.

How to Locate a Kinesiology Practitioner

When searching for a Kinesiologist, the best thing to do is to consult with a local alternative medicine professional association and obtain their members list for who practices Kinesiology in your area. You might also want to ask health practitioners you know for referrals in addition to recommendations from your friends and family members.

In your first meeting with a Kinesiology practitioner, don't hesitate to ask questions about their training, qualifications, and relevant experience. Avoid any Kinesiology practitioners who recommends that you abandon medical treatments completely that you are undergoing. These situations need to involve careful consultations with your physician.

Many symptoms related to various body ailments can be greatly relieved by Kinesiology. However, it shouldn't solely be used for diagnosing disorders. The best use of Kinesiology is to use it in combination with conventional medicine.

11

REIKI AND MASSAGE—WHAT IS IT AND HOW IT CAN HELP YOU

Basically, Reiki is healing practice that draws on spiritual energy for treating a person's aura and state of being. The literal meaning of Reiki is Universal Energy of the Life Force. This Reiki principle can be used for massage. Basically, this is the procedure of rubbing or kneading specific body parts as a type of therapy.

Many people automatically think of Reiki as a kind of massage. However, in reality, massage and Reiki are independent from one another. However, many massage therapists get Reiki healing training to enhance their massage therapy skills. Massage therapists with a Reiki background are more knowledgeable in terms of using the energy of the body to improve the client's spiritual and physical health.

Usually, a Reiki massage session starts with your head down to your body. The seven charkas, or energy centers of the body, are worked. For every specific chakra, various hand placements are used to bring the body's ability out for healing itself.

Many patients who receive Reiki massage on a regular basis have been able to improve their quality of life and have been able to develop greater pain management as well. You can distinguish Reiki massage from regular massage from how therapists don't knead or manipulate the patient's tissues or muscles.

Instead, the hands of the Reiki therapist stay very still through the entire session. This allows healing energy to be transmitted to the patient from the practitioner.

People with concerns regarding body-to-body contact don't need to worry about Reiki massage sessions. Throughout the entire Reiki massage session, the patient stays fully clothed. Skin-to-skin contact isn't needed really, and the therapist isn't likely to do anything that might cause the patient to feel uncomfortable. It is even possible to perform Reiki massage on body parts covered by a cast or bandages to send broken bones and injured muscles healing energy.

Reiki massage can be used to treat various ailments like tension, lock jaw or TMJ, pain, injuries, stress, and muscle pain, along with many other kinds of medical conditions.

Mikau Usui, a Japanese doctor, was the one who discovered the Reiki principle and applied this to therapeutic procedures. Reiki principles, however, have been in existence for thousands of years, especially in ancient Tibet. Animals and plants, in addition to people, can be treated by Reiki practitioners.

Anybody with an open mind when it comes to spiritual healing can learn the Reiki craft. Students in Reiki classes study the various meditation and hand placements that might help with healing patients. Students study how the seven charkas of the body can be manipulated to bring healing for different ailments and illnesses.

It is believed that Reiki sessions are completely safe since they don't cause any side effects or injuries to the patient. During a session, different sensations might be felt, which may range from a tingling sensation to a warm feeling.

Reiki healing might even be conducted over a long distance. A Reiki Master might send healing energies anyplace in the world.

However, Reiki does require a big opening of one's mind by the patient as well as the practitioner. Usually, the massage is used for reinforcing Reiki healing, and for helping the patient be able to ease into his healing process. Music is often involved in a Reiki healing session to amplify releasing healing energies.

What's great about Reiki is it doesn't treat the illness. Instead, it treats what caused the illness in the first place. The healing imparted by Reiki applies to all levels of one's state of being. Therefore, the form of treatment isn't merely superficial. Among the many who benefit from Reiki massage sessions include individuals who have problems relaxing, adults and children with ADHD, individuals with emotional and mental problems, and individuals with various body and mind disorders.

It also has been observed that Reiki helps individuals change unwanted and old habits like smoking. It has even been seen that Reiki helps with relieving strains, sprains, headaches, flu, and colds.

Reiki, however, should not be viewed as a complete substitute of conventional healing methods. Reiki, at best, can be used for supplementing most medical treatments for its best effect. If you want to learn more about Reiki, ask local alternative medicine organizations and practitioners for more information.

12

SPORTS MASSAGE 101: KEY POINTS YOU SHOULD KNOW

The Basics of Sports Massage

Throughout history, people have been utilizing the healing powers of massage. The history of massage can be traced back for thousands of years, and it can be found in several different cultures. That said, massages have only recently begun to be embraced by modern medicine. Sports massage is one type of treatment that's becoming particularly popular.

What can sports massage do?

Like with any type of massage, the goal of sports massage is to improve the overall health of the patient. However, sports massage also focuses on improving the athlete's natural abilities Techniques that will strengthen their performance and improve their muscle recovery are employed. An increasing number of athletes are beginning to rely on the power of spots massage. It allows them to recover very quickly and gives them significant improvements to their performance.

Sports massage uses the power of anatomy and physiology to improve the strength of the skeletal and muscular systems. Massage practitioners need a great deal of training to be able to employ these message techniques effectively.

A good masseuse uses their understanding of the human body to strengthen and heal an athlete.

When training for a sport, the goal is to improve an athlete's abilities. They can be a stronger competitor if they work to improve their stamina, speed, agility, strength, and skill. Many athletes push their bodies to the limit as they work to become stronger. Unfortunately, this level of training often leads to the body becoming overworked.

This kind of abuse can hinder an athlete's performance over time. It can damage their bones and muscles and can lead to several ailments. It also puts athletes at risk for injury and trauma. This is the primary reason why the injury rate for athletes is so high.

The body is more than capable of recovering from this abuse, but continuous sports training makes it hard for the body to heal in the way it needs to. Athletes can't afford to give their body the break it needs, because they need to keep on training. Therefore, sports massage can be so helpful. It allows athletes to recover from the challenges of their training at a rapid rate and gives them a chance to properly recuperate.

Why a sports massage can benefit you

When a sports massage is carried out by a well-trained practitioner, it can be incredibly effective. It will restore the muscles while easing tension at the same time. Massage can significantly reduce the rate of injury, especially when it comes to injuries that have to do with muscle overuse. When bones and muscles are frequently subjected to intense activity, the joints become stressed. There is also a great deal of stress placed on the muscles, tendons, and ligaments.

In many cases, these problems go unnoticed until they're severe enough to cause significant problems for the athlete. Thankfully, a qualified sport massage practitioner can detect these problems right away. They can find and treat the issue before it becomes a major problem.

When it comes to sports massage, what should you watch out for?

In most cases, sports massage will only benefit athletes. However, there are a few situations in which sports massage can be detrimental. There are certain types of injuries that can be worsened by massage techniques. Avoid sports massage under these circumstances:

- When you have an open wound or contusion, or other acute injury
- When you have a fever of more than 100 degrees.
- If you're experiencing blood vessel abnormalities, like phlebitis, thrombosis, or varicose veins.
- If you suffer from hemophilia.
- If you have an infectious disease, like herpes, a fungal infection, or a virus
- If you have a cyst or tumor

If you're dealing with one of these issues, talk to a doctor before visiting a sports massage practitioner. You don't want to get a sports massage if it will make matters worse. Even if the massage practitioner is aware of the issue, it can cause problems.

In most cases, sports massage can do a great deal to improve an athlete's health and safety. It can be hugely beneficial and has very few drawbacks. It's something worth trying.

If you'd like to find additional information on sports massage, talk to a sports specialist or health practitioner. They'll be able to give you the information you need and can refer you to a licensed practitioner.

13

PET MASSAGE—THERAPY FOR YOUR PETS

Touch therapy has been acclaimed to be among the best energy boosters and vitamins that any creature can have for a very long time.

So, it really isn't a surprise that so many animal lovers strongly recommend massage therapy or touch therapy for their pets. Many individuals don't realize it; however, massage is among the best therapies you can give your pet.

Pet massage can do incredible things for animals' circulatory systems. It may cause significant changes to blood circulation, which eradicates poisonous substances from the body and nourishes the cells.

What people provide their pets when they take them to get a massage is physiologically very healthful. Numerous cases have shown how massage for animals offers very positive results.

The explanation provided is living creatures have been created and have energy fields that surround them. The energies radiate from inside and extend from the body two to four inches and outline the body and head. Auras, have they have been exposed, are formed and often some people can see them.

People for a very long time have always held the belief that humans are the only ones who possess an energy field or aura. What so many are not aware of is that animals, plants and even objects can have auras as well.

These energy fields, if the conditions are right, can be seen by the human eye. They reflect the state of physical health.

As a result, according to experts, individuals who can see and feel energies can deeply control or influence the field via massage.

When energy fields overlap, it can bring positive effects with it, especially when an individual massages or touches another living creature. The positive energy of the person gets transmitted over to the living creature. This creates a fresher energy field. A cure is therefore likely.

This is why so many pet lovers now are strongly recommending pet massages to increase their resistance to disease and give a boost to life expectancy.

Anyway, massage for pets don't make just pets feel better. Massage for pets may bring positive effects to humans also.

For example, massage can help to reduce or maintain your blood pressure. Massage for pets lets you release specific negative energies. Therefore, it releases energies that are negative and radiating from inside.

Surveys, in fact, show that almost 85% of individuals with pets who give them massages on a frequent basis are not prone to getting diseases or illnesses.

Massage for pets isn't considered an extra activity that they do. It's more like a necessity for further nourishing the health of your pet.

Watch how pets, such as dogs and cats, respond to a massage. They woof and purr whenever their owners massage their back or stroke their head.

In order for you to begin promoting optimum health for your pet, you need to learn how to give your pets influential strokes and allow positive reactions to be created for their owners. This is how you do it:

Start with the shoulders

Massage for pets may influence the quick reflexes of the animal directly in addition to releasing stress and tension that gets buried in the shoulders. According to experts, massage for pets can be good for them, particularly when they really need it.

Starting with the shoulders is best thing to do. Animal shoulders, just like humans, are the best area to target for releasing stress and tension. The key is placing pressure on each movement. That way, your pet can catch some of your body's positive energy.

Stroking time

Just stroke the body of your pet. Work from his shoulders down to his tail. This type of friction that gets created from directly touching the fur of your pet can help to stimulate his blood circulation in addition to influencing his behavior.

What most people don't realize is that one main reason why pets get excited and irritable at times is due to pets getting anxious or bored.

Since your pet can't verbally express his sentiments or feelings, he takes whatever actions he can to convey whatever message he wants to reveal to you.

Pets, like humans, can be relaxed and relieved after they've felt their owner's touch and heard their voice as well. Massage for pets isn't only therapy. In addition, it can be considered the ideal way of creating and maintaining a bond with your pet.

Massage for pets may indeed be the ultimate health and energy booster. Because they are unable to do anything physically to relieve tension and stress, which animals are known to get, massage for pets might just be the answer.

14

YOU CAN BE A MASSAGE THERAPIST YOURSELF—HERE'S HOW

The most powerful tool for pain relief that nurses have available to them is pain medication. However, it isn't the only option. There are other nursing activities that are non-pharmacological in nature that can help with relieving a patient's pain and come with only low risk.

These measures may not be a complete substitute for medication. However, they might be all that is appropriate or needed for relieving painful episodes that just last just minutes or even seconds.

In situations of severe pain lasting for hours or days, often the most effective method for relieving pain involves combining medications with non- pharmacological interventions.

The gain control theory on pain posits that when the fibers transmitting non- painful sensations are stimulated, it can decrease or block pain impulses from being transmitted.

There are several pain relief non-pharmacological strategies that have their basis in this theory, including using cold and heat while rubbing the skin.

Massage, which involves a generalized stimulation of the body's skin, frequently focuses on the shoulders and back. Massages don't specifically stimulate non-pain receptors that are in the pain receptor field. However, its descending control system can still leave an impact.

Comfort is also promoted by massage since it is very helpful in getting the body's muscles to relax.

Therefore, with massage growing in popularity due its many positive effects, many individuals are inspired to study massage therapy. By doing this, they can provide other people with positive effects and enjoy their own positive effects all at the very same time.

Massage therapists, through this activity, can help relieve the discomfort and pain experienced by other people. Therefore, most massage therapists view this to be an invigorating experience. Helping another person can be a great feeling when you can provide them with comfort and nourishment.

However, it isn't easy to become a massage therapist. Before you decide to become one, it's very important for you to know what is involved.

Here are some useful tips to help you get started with becoming a massage therapist. They are factors that can help you determine whether massage therapy can benefit you or not.

Evaluate yourself

One of the main keys for becoming a great massage therapist is analyzing your potential of being able to provide people in pain with support and comfort. You won't ever be effective as a massage therapist if you can't offer relaxation and comfort voluntarily.

Massage therapy is just a regular non-pharmacological method for relieving the pain and discomfort that another person is experiencing. It has more to do with giving another person some of your energy to lighten their burden. Therefore, if you don't think you will be able to give some of yourself to others, it probably isn't a good option for you to become a massage therapist.

Becoming a massage therapist also doesn't require a lot of supervision. Therefore, it's best if you can work on your own and not need to be supervised all of the time.

Learning effective communication skills is also very important. This is the main tool you will use when reaching out to clients and speaking with them.

Educate yourself

It isn't a joke to become a massage therapist. It involves more than just pain relief and physical relaxation. It's more about applying the correct principles and techniques to relieve pain effectively for people suffering from discomfort and pain.

You should receive comprehensive massage therapist training before becoming one. This will enable you to apply the best techniques and enable you to become a practicing message therapist for your local community.

Do your homework

Before you choose to be a massage therapist, it's critical that you know what you're getting yourself into first. There are numerous kinds of massage. It requires plenty of dedication and time to learn them. Do research on massage therapy. For each kind of therapy, learn the fundamentals. To make good decisions, it is vital that you have the right information.

Determine what the local requirements are for massage practice.

Before you will be able to practice massage therapy, you will need to follow and obtain certain requirements first. Identify what your area's specific requirements are. Remember that requirements will vary from one state to the next.

Helping other people of course is a rewarding experience all on its own. However, it's even more invigorating to help others with massage therapy. Becoming a massage therapist isn't just a career or skill. It is a vocation that involves giving part of yourself to help ease the pain of others.

How to Run a Massage Practice Using These 6 Easy Steps

With massage therapy being so efficient and feasible, more and more individuals are beginning to establish their massage practice as their chosen form of business.

Massage therapy, since the ancient days, has been used for curing different diseases. Massage therapists back then had no to little formal training when it came to practicing massage. As civilization kept developing and the industry was proliferated with technology, the practice of massage has developed into a form of business that is more professional. It now focuses on administering massage practice and proper training.

Today running a massage practice is thought to be among the more rewarding of all ventures. Not only is it monetarily rewarding, it is also psychosocially and physically rewarding as well.

So, if you happen to be considering starting a massage therapy practice to help build your future, here are some tips for how to run a massage practice.

Remember that before you can be a massage therapist, there are many massage therapy principles and techniques that you will need to learn first.

Self-assessment

A massage practice isn't for everyone. There are people who would love to run a massage practice, but discover they aren't fit for operating this type of business.

Just as many writers are born instead of made, massage therapists have to be created and talent for it isn't innate. Some innate qualities, however, are needed for facilitating the learning process and applying the principles and theories of massage therapy.

Therefore, before starting a massage practice, be sure to first thoroughly evaluate yourself first to ensure you have necessary qualities for running this kind of business.

For example, massage practices need people who can efficiently work under minimum supervision, are compassionate, have good communication skills and are affable.

If you have these characteristics, it will make running a massage practice a lot easier for you.

Select your field

There isn't just one field that massage practice focuses on. It involves a mixture of various types of massage all rolled into one.

The best thing is knowing you can do all the different kinds. However, specializing in one kind of massage is the best thing to do. Try identifying the kind of massage you would be best suited to work with. You could choose Swedish massage, deep tissue massage, etc.

Another thing you could do is concentrate in a certain field of specialization like pregnancy massage or animal massage.

Wisely choose your service

You can conduct your massage practice at a workspace or at home. Review the pros and cons for each of these options. Try to determine which kind of business will work the best for you.

Get trained

Before you can begin running your own massage practice, it's critical that you get all the necessary training first. Remember that today's massage practices focus on high quality services and professionalism.

Therefore, you want to make sure you get the most suitable and best training so that you can effectively deliver your services. If you are properly trained in massage therapy before you start your massage practice, you'll have the ability to provide your services as principally and theoretically correct as possible. Also, massage therapy training will you an expert in the field of massage.

Complete all the necessary requirements

With massage practices becoming so popular, many individuals thought they would be able to easily start their message therapy businesses without a lot of hassle.

The government currently has certain requirements and imposed rules before someone can run a massage practice. The requirements vary from one state to the next. Therefore, it is very important for you to know what is required by your state so you can complete all the necessary steps before starting your massage business.

Lead a healthy life

Massage therapy does tend to drain a person's energy who performs massages. Therefore, the best thing to do is get regular energy boosts and follow a healthy routine.

Regular exercise and consuming a balanced diet can help a massage therapist lead a healthy life as well as promote health and wellness for others via massage therapy.

It can be easy to run a massage practice. There are just some factors you need to consider that will allow you to begin running a massage practice.

Remember that massage practice must deal with other things besides delivering quality services and the correct administration of curative measures. However, it isn't necessary to invest in other kinds of tangible items like other kinds of businesses do. Therefore, the best thing to do is to focus on those factors and get them developed so that you can effectively manage your massage practice.

ABOUT THE AUTHOR

Hermilando "Ingming" Duque Aberia is a social development worker by training and profession. He worked in international development agencies like the United Nations Conference on Trade and Development, United Nations Development Program, International Labor Organization and Asian Development Bank. He holds a master's degree in Development Management from the Makati-based Asian Institute of Management.

He also contributes articles once a week to The Manila Times as OpEd columnist.

He also dabbles as administrator for several websites, such as:

- IngmingAberia.com and www.Ingming.Aberia.us (personal blog);

- GlobalPinoyHomes.com (a real estate property listing website);

- IMInstitute.org (information site for online marketers);

- HealthBeautyAndFitness.today (a health and fitness blog).